THE OTHER SIDE

LIVING WITH MULTIPLE SCLEROSIS

Janet M. Cogoli, M.D.

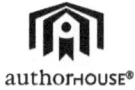

authorHOUSE®

AuthorHouse™
1663 Liberty Drive
Bloomington, IN 47403
www.authorhouse.com
Phone: 1-800-839-8640

First published by AuthorHouse 07/14/2011

ISBN: 978-1-4634-0808-4 (sc)
ISBN: 978-1-4634-0809-1 (ebk)

Library of Congress Control Number: 2011908711

Printed in the United States of America

Any people depicted in stock imagery provided by Thinkstock are models, and such images are being used for illustrative purposes only. Certain stock imagery © Thinkstock.

This book is printed on acid-free paper.

DEDICATION

This book is for my deceased parents,
Shirley Rose (Ledoux) Cogoli and
William Joseph Cogoli.
To them, I owe all good things in life.

To my deceased brother,
William Edward Cogoli,
who spoke my language, was my adventurous partner,
and always reminded me of life's realities.

To my many doctors, teachers, and professors,
who have always tried their best.

To my CNAs,
who have been with me in both good times and bad
and have helped me in so many ways.

To all of the MS patients whom I have met in my practice and to
the many others with MS nationwide, as well as their families.

My love to you all:
Without your presence, I could not have enjoyed life as I have.

TABLE OF CONTENTS

PREFACE

This is an account of my private and professional experience with multiple sclerosis. It has been thirty years since I was diagnosed. I am a physician and a patient. I have studied it, treated it, suffered with it, and now I would like to empathize with others also affected by this disease. I hope that this book will improve understanding by other professionals. I will be writing this as an autobiography, though I acknowledge that everyone has his or her own unique, important story.

I am a physiatrist (physical medicine and rehabilitation), not a neurologist, and do not mean this to be a textbook. So, some of the information herein has not been researched extensively nor written with this in mind. Please critique it kindly.

My specialty deals with helping people reach their maximum functional potential, despite physical disability. There are a number of professionals involved in the rehabilitation process, including physical therapists, occupational therapists, speech therapists, social workers, rehab nurses, and neuropsychologists. Doctors such as orthopedic surgeons, internists, and urologists are also team members.

The physiatrist is an M.D. or a D.O. who coordinates the patient's care with the therapists' roles. The physiatrist must be familiar with the medical and social needs of the patient. Since negotiation with insurance companies is usually necessary, the physiatrist must also be the patient's advocate.

Please enjoy and think of this book as a friendly conversation between you and me. It is written for you, your family, and interested others. Again, this is not a textbook; there are many good ones already published.

The book begins with a definition of multiple sclerosis, and then a section on neuroanatomy follows. The neuroanatomy has been simplified in order to be easily understood. It should help with the explanations of multiple sclerosis symptoms.

The next part will be a history detailing the lives of my grandfather and my parents. I hope that you find this interesting and of value. These people have given me inspiration, courage, and hope. Then I'll describe my personal history and the problems I've had with multiple sclerosis.

In the contents, I'll address some of the more common symptoms and give explanations for their occurrence, as well as the ways of dealing with them that have been successful for others and me.

This section will also include both medicines that are currently in use and others being investigated.

DEFINITION OF MULTIPLE SCLEROSIS

Multiple Sclerosis (MS, hereafter used interchangeably) is an autoimmune disease affecting the central nervous system (CNS). Autoimmune is a term that refers to antibodies produced against the host itself, and while it has been proven that the autoimmune system is involved, exactly how is not yet known. Attempts to find an infectious agent that might be involved...alas, they have failed. In fact, there is still too much about multiple sclerosis which is not yet understood, but we do know that it is not contagious, is more common in women than men, and is also more common in people who live north of the equator. It may be inherited and at this time much genetic research is being done. There might also be an environmental factor involved.

In the United States, multiple sclerosis has an incidence of 400,000, with 200 new diagnoses made each week. The total number of cases in the world is about 2.5 million. MS is known to occur in all age groups, from young children to the elderly.

Myelin is the very important structure that will be addressed throughout this book. It is a coating on the nerves of the CNS which acts like insulation on electrical wires. It permits rapid, efficient signal transmission through the nerves, which, in turn, results in smooth, coordinated movement. This is accomplished involuntarily and is often taken for granted. Breaks in the insulation or areas of demyelination result in interrupted signal transmission and in the many symptoms seen in multiple sclerosis.

It is also worth mentioning the four different courses that are seen in multiple sclerosis. The *benign course* consists of a remitting pattern, with very long periods of stability. The *relapsing-remitting course* usually involves many periodic attacks, followed by remissions (recovery). This results in slow but steadily progressive disability. This is also called secondary progressive. The ***chronic-progressive course***, usually seen in older people, consists of steady progression without remission and resultant severe disability. Finally, for those few with a ***malignant course***, total disability and death occur within months.

NEUROANATOMY

The CNS consists of the **brain**, or better referred to as the **cerebrum**, which is the major control center for thought, movement, and sensation. Behind the brain is the **cerebellum**, responsible for coordinating movements of the extremities, and also for balance—especially, but not only—with walking. The **brainstem** is beneath the cerebrum and the cerebellum and is responsible for controlling vital functions such as the heart, lungs, and also eye movement.

Beneath all of these is the **spinal cord**, which is like a huge telephone pole, insulated by myelin. It functions by quickly and efficiently transmitting signals from the brain to and from the body below.

Then we have the nervous system, located in the extremities, known as the **peripheral nervous system**, or PNS. The extremities may be affected by weakness or other symptoms in multiple sclerosis not because of problems in the PNS itself but because of problems in the brain or spinal cord, resulting in interrupted signal transmission.

Finally, there is the **autonomic nervous system**, which automatically controls the bowel, heart rate, and other necessary functions on its own. It indirectly communicates with the CNS.

FOREBEARS' HISTORY

This story actually begins at a time far before my appearance. It is an interesting account of some lives which, I hope, will impress you by the courageousness of the characters. I would like it to be an example of perseverance, which I will also try to achieve with this writing. The story starts with the history of my Italian grandfather as told to me by my father.

Giovanni Battista Cogoli, my grandfather, was born in 1885 in Pordenone, Italy. This city is in northern Italy, about forty miles northeast of Venice. Battista's (Italians often go by their middle names) father, Luigi, was well established as a musician and a superintendent of the shipping department in the city's leading textile mill. In time, however, Luigi was offered and accepted a better position with a firm in South America.

After establishing himself there, Luigi sent for his son and wife, who were still in Italy. They boarded a ship in 1894 with their destination being Montevideo, Uruguay. Like many other Europeans at that time, they were immigrants seeking a better life and better jobs. As fate would have it, shortly after their arrival in the port of Santos, Brazil, they received word of Luigi's death.

Now they were grief-stricken and stranded in a foreign land. They felt lucky, however, when they learned that the *Cafaro*, the ship on which they had traveled to South America, went on to sink only two days after she had left them at the port of Santos.

After working in Santos for about one year, Battista, his mother, and some Italian friends whom they had met traveled by train to São Paulo, where they found even better jobs. There they stayed for about six months. Then they heard of a big plantation where the workers were mostly Italian and were paid higher wages. So off they went by train, for twelve hours, until they reached Jaboticabal, and then traveled fifteen more miles by horse to Monte Alto de Jaboticabal. So now, at the age of ten, Battista secured work on the plantation. He was paid about seven dollars each month, including room and board.

Six years later, his mother died. At sixteen, he was alone and terrified in a new land with few friends. Yet, he was able to earn a man's wages, had learned to read and write Portuguese well, and had mastered his mathematics. The situation was not altogether hopeless. Every night, he was able to attend school on the plantation and paid the teacher three dollars each month.

His hard work paid off because his boss, who had acquired a new plot of land on the Brazilian frontier, put him in charge of cultivation of this land. He was assigned two men and a woman to help him with the cultivation. Necessary tools were sent to the new location by mule train.

The foursome began to walk to reach their destination from about seven o'clock every morning until it was too dark to see. They would go to sleep next to a fire, which was kept ablaze to scare wild animals away. They also had a dog, which must have saved them one night, because the next morning they saw paw prints of a jaguar circling their campsite.

After reaching the location where they would build their home, their first job was to construct a log cabin. They used a few simple tools which they had brought along. These included only a saw, an ax, and a drill. With hard work, their house was soon completed.

Next, they needed to clear the land for cultivation. After two long months, they had cut down many trees. Now they knew that the only way to clear the land was to burn their way through the trees. According to the law, they needed to clear a border of twelve feet around the trees and then burn it. This they successfully did. They set the fire against the wind. Luckily, all went well. After the first big rain, the land was ready for planting, on which they grew corn, rice, coffee, and sugarcane.

One day, Pietro, a professional jaguar hunter, invited Battista on a hunt. Again, luck was with Battista and he was able to kill the jaguar as it was descending from a large tree. My grandfather loved to tell of his adventure. He could recall all of the details many years later. Of course, his Italian needed to be translated by his wife, who had learned English by attending night school.

His story went like this: "The big cat glared at me with round, black eyes…black as coal and huge, dark pupils. Both of its ears were tilted back almost flat and the whiskers moved with its mouth, from which came loud, threatening snarls and growls, as if he was coming to get me! Its face had a frightening, sickening grin. The muscles of its shoulders, arms, and chest bulged out from beneath its brilliant gold coat with spots of black. I raised my gun up to my shoulder, aimed it, pulled the trigger, and pow!!!

"I remember the deafening sound of the gun and how the small animals in the underbrush ran away to seek shelter. I also saw monkeys swinging from nearby treetops to those more distant. They screamed so loud! I witnessed that, slowly, the big cat's claws loosened their hold from the soft tree bark they had gripped tightly. Droplets of blood fell to the ground. The cat slipped limply to the ground, too. I saw that there was a round mark on its chest rimmed with blood. I remember, then, wiping the sweat from my forehead with a very tired arm. My heart was pounding.

"Now all was strangely quiet in the forest. I looked down at the cat with feelings of guilt and sadness. It was truly a magnificent animal, but no longer would it terrorize the local people. For this reason, I was able to justify my feelings of guilt."

As a gift of gratitude, Battista was given fifteen dollars by Pietro. He returned to his plantation, where he had worked so hard to get the crops off to a good start, but was greeted with the news that one of his helpers had caught yellow fever and been taken by another to the city. The other helper who had been left alone had been kidnapped. Battista armed himself and with a friend, went in pursuit of the criminal, but he was too late.

Now, unable to take care of the plantation by himself, he had to sell what he could. He decided that the best option was to return to the city. Maybe he would be able to find some work there. Luckily, he met some people who would become good friends. One of his new friends was Salvatore Rossi.

By now, you must be wondering what the point is with this story, but my message is meant to convey how far courage can take a person. There is more to the story, and this is very important.

Salvatore Rossi became a trusted friend of Battista's. He had relatives in the United States of America and often told Battista of the opportunities he had heard about in the new country. Both felt that they could perhaps find some of those good opportunities in America. So, they left Santos and arrived by ship in New York on the fourth of July, 1905. Salvatore had relatives in Worcester, Massachusetts. They boarded a train and arrived in Worcester from Boston.

Battista got his first job in America on September 20, 1905, in Worcester, at the Graton & Knight Manufacturing Company. In 1907, he married Maria Zuppo, the niece of one of the men he had known very well in South America. Mary, my grandmother, had come to America from Calabria, southern Italy, with her mother at the tender age of five.

Battista went to become the father of eight children, one of whom was my father, William. In 1922, he became a naturalized citizen of the United States of America. In his later years, Battista still enjoyed planting; his true passion was planting peach trees. He also had a route through the woods, where he would take my dad. He knew the tree where the best mushrooms grew. He also knew the poisonous ones to avoid. He grew beautiful grapes and made fine, red wine. As he had in Brazil, he loved growing trees and edible plants.

As you can see, Battista was someone who rose to the occasion with courage whenever presented with problems. He turned them into actions to survive and opportunities to better himself.

This is also what I am trying to do with this book, and I hope I will succeed. I also hope to encourage others who struggle to know that their struggle is important, albeit often very difficult and with many unknown consequences.

I think that one must personally experience a difficult physical problem so as to fully understand how hard it can be to deal with. Those of us who have contended with disability also realize how others sometimes seem to take so much for granted.

Of course, how we are able to carry on depends on the situation at hand. Nevertheless, I want to encourage others to not give up the struggle. Even a smile, though difficult at times, will change others' attitudes in a positive way, which will be of benefit and thus make life easier.

FAMILY HISTORY

I'll continue first with the story of my immediate family. Though by heritage I am Italian and French, I remember my father telling me that his father had always told his kids—when asked if he would teach them Italian—that they were in America and English was the language they needed to learn.

My grandfather was proud of his citizenship and knew that his children would have to master the language and use it properly, in order to secure jobs and be accepted. So, he never taught them and, therefore, my father and I never learned conversational Italian. My French is better only because of the courses I've taken in high school and college. French was the popular language at that time. Anyway, don't worry: this book is written in English, and I think my grandfather would have approved it.

My mother's father came to this country by way of Canada and worked as a train engineer. Her mother traveled to the States from Italy. Her parents instilled in my mother the appropriateness of hard work and of always trying her best, which she followed by providing me with a good home and an excellent education.

As a young child, I remember walking with her up to the center of town, practically every day, and buying a new book as soon as I finished the one that I had been reading. She encouraged me to keep this up. I remember reading those books to my neighbor. She and my dad always helped with homework when I was in need of help. They always found the time and continually stressed the importance of doing my best.

My mother was a secretary, a volunteer with the American Red Cross, a lab assistant, and even worked in the high-school cafeteria at one time. She took the bus to work every day (few women drove cars in those days), in all kinds of weather, and never complained.

At the age of 75, she died a painful death due to peritoneal cancer, during which course she was also afflicted with renal failure and abdominal obstruction, and then a heart attack and pneumonia—all in all, an unspeakably horrific demise. I never got to help her endure chemo. I intended to, but we didn't get a chance. I meant to help her exit from this world just as she had helped me enter it.

One winter day, just after I had left from visiting her in the hospital, I was told that she had coded and didn't survive. It was a lot quicker than I thought it would be. I guess I was too hopeful and in denial of what I already knew would happen. It was her time. At least, she wouldn't suffer anymore. I didn't agree to an autopsy. After all, we knew what had happened; it was too personal and it hurt too much. We called for the hospital priest. I needed faith at that time, not science.

My father also worked very hard to provide us with a good home and education. He was the first child in his family with a college education. He graduated from Worcester Polytechnic Institute and became a mechanical engineer. Then he joined the Navy and served in World War II. His first job was with Rockwood Sprinkler Company in Worcester. That is where he met my mother. He traveled to many locations measuring buildings for sprinkler systems.

He helped to build our house in 1952. He even landscaped the yard. After the job in Worcester, he worked for American Optical in Putnam, Connecticut. I remember him getting up at five every morning to begin the long drive. He worked there until he was laid off in 1982, the year I graduated from medical school and was married.

My parents were determined that my brother and I would have a good college education. But those were the years of the Vietnam War and we all prayed that my brother would escape the draft. I remember always anxiously hoping that his number would never be called. I listened to the radio each morning, hearing about the war's numerous casualties. Thank God his number was *not* called; our prayers had been answered.

My parents had given enough. After all, they had lived through the Depression, been raised by hard-working immigrants, and served in World War II. They were members of that great generation. I never heard them complain, but went on sacrificing and on giving both of us a good education.

We were living the dream of the 1950s, whereby all parents wanted better lives for their children than what they had experienced. We were expected to appreciate the opportunities that had been given us. My father always told me that I could become whatever I wanted; I just had to work hard and he was sure that I would. My parents had a lot of faith in me. Luck was with me.

My father died at the age of 81, of metastatic colon cancer. He died at home. It was not easy. He underwent surgery, but the cancer had spread to a lymph node and the chemotherapy ceased to work. He was a hospice patient at the time of his death. I held his hand until he took his last breath and said the eulogy at his funeral. I prayed for him. I *still* pray for him, my mother, and my brother every day.

My brother died at the age of 54, a real shock to everyone. I'm not sure what happened to him. His youngest son found him dead one morning. It was utterly tragic. Emphysema might have been the cause; that's my guess. His doctor had diagnosed him with COPD. As hard as he tried, he couldn't quit the habit of smoking. Too many guys at work also smoked, he would tell me.

I had tried to help him for quite a few years, but I guess I failed. Smoking was a hard addiction to beat. So, I read at his funeral mass. It was the least I could do.

PERSONAL HISTORY

Now it's on to *my* story:

I chose to become a physician. I used to be an amateur artist and, at first, wanted to become a plastic surgeon. I thought that this would be a good profession for a woman. I wanted to be independent and responsible for myself. My parents' habit of working hard to achieve had been handed down to me and I like to think that I've inherited my courage from *all* of the people I've described for you. So I worked very hard to get to that point in my life. I knew that it would be difficult to qualify for medical school, but I had persevered to reach my dream. *I* had my life ***all*** planned. It was to be a real fast track to success and I saw no problems in the way. I'll describe what was going on, so please bear with me, for this is a long story, as I'm sure many of you with MS will understand, having experienced similar issues yourselves.

I graduated from public high school in three years and was accepted at Mount Holyoke College. I chose a major in Biochemistry. It was a difficult though fascinating subject. When I took my oral exam, I remember having to explain how life on Earth might have begun. Of course, I had to use what I had learned so far in Biochemistry. It was a big challenge, the biggest I had experienced so far.

I managed to graduate magna cum laude in 1978, was elected to Phi Beta Kappa, Sigma Xi Scientific Research Society, and carried a 4.0 grade point average. I was also a Mary Lyon Scholar (named after the woman who founded this first college for women) and a Sarah Williston Scholar.

I was accepted at the University of Massachusetts Medical School in 1978 and spent the following summer doing cardiovascular research in the lab of the professor who later would teach cardiac physiology to my medical-school class. With his guidance, I published my first research paper.

My world was still perfect. I had great plans for the future…but I was not—and I mean **NOT**—prepared for what was to come; in fact, I would never have imagined it. I mean, not me! I might have pipetted too many dangerous chemicals and dealt with too much radioactive Adenosine Triphosphate (ATP), but I *never* saw this coming.

My MS began in 1979, when I was in my second year of medical school. I was twenty-one. In November, strange things began to happen. As I remember, the left, lower eyelid and the left side of my face began twitching such that it was a bother as I tried to read. This persisted and was difficult to ignore, since reading at this time was what I needed to constantly do. In addition, I developed a left, sixth-nerve palsy, resulting in a lot of trouble with double vision. This led to my first experience with work-ups, including a spinal tap and a CT.

These tests were normal and luckily those symptoms resolved completely. So, life was *still* good. After all, these were problems that came and then went away. I remember that it was a little while later when I experienced some unsteady walking at a Christmas party which one of my classmates was hosting, but I ignored this problem. After all, I wanted to be okay like everyone else. I was too busy to attach any significance to it; besides, I didn't yet understand its importance.

In the spring of 1980, one morning I suffered severe nausea, followed by what felt like a fluid level in my head, which would slosh whenever I moved my head, increasing the nausea. I remember lying down and just hoping that the sensation would go away. I was miserable and paralyzed by fear of what could be happening. I learned later that this was severe vertigo. Significant fatigue also started, and was much worse that I had *ever* known.

I remember, then, having a spinal angiogram. Several CTs followed. Then, severe gait ataxia appeared and I was treated with Prednisone. The symptoms resolved over several months. Around that time, I remember going to Boston for help with the diagnosis. I was, again, having a lot of trouble walking. The hospital halls felt as though they were *way* too long. The neurologist examined me and studied the CTs that I had brought with me. I remember hoping that he would not see a tumor. To this day, I still hate it when doctors look at CTs and MRIs of my brain.

It is too personal. In a way, I feel embarrassed and violated. After all, regardless of the pathology that the scans demonstrate, I'm still me, and there's still a lot about my mind and soul that they will *never* know!

Anyway, the neurologist came out to the waiting room that day and announced that I had multiple sclerosis. My parents were devastated. I remember the look on their faces. The neurologist didn't seem too concerned. I never saw that doctor again; he had, after all, merely been the bearer of some very bad news. I was, nevertheless, glad that it wasn't a brainstem tumor; that's what I had feared. I guess I was still young and hopeful and inexperienced.

The disease convinced me to take some time off. I had never experienced so much fatigue. Even walking seemed to take all my strength. I missed all of my final exams and would eventually have to catch up with my class, so I spent the summer studying and taking around ten exams. Ah, medical school demands so much from one...! I remember sleeping *a lot* that summer. I couldn't help it. Dad would call me from Connecticut, practically every day, to see how I was.

My clinical rotations were quite challenging. The dean suggested that I take a year off, but I saw no reason to do so. I didn't want to give up and feel defeated; I *had* to go on. Walking through the hospital halls was difficult because they were bright white and this bothered my eyes. It was painful, as if I were walking outside in glaring sunlight. Something was still wrong with the vision, but I wanted to continue.

November of 1981 found me struggling with a right optic neuritis and an internuclear opthalmoplegia. Again, I was treated with oral Prednisone and the symptoms improved. It was about this time that a medical-school professor of neurology listened to my history and performed an EMG on me. She determined that I had a left facial myokymia, and taken together with my course so far, she agreed that the diagnosis was multiple sclerosis.

Despite these problems, I was able to successfully complete my clinical rotations. I graduated in June of 1982 with my class. Life was problematic but still good. To look at me then, one would never have known that I had multiple sclerosis.

Thus far, I had been lucky. I kept hoping that it would be a benign course, but the neurologist at my medical school who had diagnosed the facial myokymia advised me to give up my dream of plastic surgery as a career, in case I developed a tremor in my hands. She suggested, instead, a specialty called physical medicine and rehabilitation, which was offered at the Mayo Clinic, where she had trained in neurology. Imagine that…! How could a tremor change one's life? I was disappointed but clearly still driven.

I heeded her advice and off I went to Rochester, Minnesota. In July of 1982, I began my residency at the Mayo Clinic. Unfortunately, I also began to suffer with painful tingling of both feet. This was followed, in August, 1982, by urinary retention. I was treated with oral Prednisone.

In March of 1984, an acute onset of nystagmus occurred and treatment again with Prednisone for another month. During the same month, internuclear opthalmoplegia recurred but resolved over two months.

In April of 1984, I had difficulty with control of the left upper and left lower extremities. There was also decreased sensation of the right side of the body. I was treated with Prednisone for two weeks. The symptoms went on to improve.

In June of 1984, blind spots occurred in the left eye, resulting in a paracentral scotoma. These symptoms and signs also resolved completely.

In July of 1984, I experienced numbness in the left arm and hand, which gradually spread to involve the torso over a few days. I could not manipulate a pen properly with the left hand. There was also a pressure-like feeling along the upper part of the extremity. Oral Prednisone was again begun at 100 mg and decreased to 8 mg in late July. This time, there was no improvement.

I was, then, admitted to Mayo Clinic–affiliated Methodist Hospital with complaints of numbness of the left side of the body and inability to control the left hand, something which had been bothering me for three weeks. I could not write. Work-up at this time included another spinal tap.

The tap revealed oligoclonal bands and increased protein. A median somatosensory–evoked potential on the left was abnormal at the neck. In addition, there was a visual-evoked response, which was interpreted as showing that there was minimal slowing of conduction latencies, with stimulation of both the right and the left eye. An MRI was also done.

Now the diagnosis was definitely multiple sclerosis. For the first time, IV steroids were to be given. The dose was 1000 mg per day for five days. I was told that, *if* I were to get better, the steroids would hasten the recovery…but there was *no* guarantee. All would depend on how much inflammation was present.

For the first time, the test results clearly showed that this disease was multiple sclerosis. Now I had to admit it again: it would NOT go away. It was rather sad. My denial could no longer go on…but life does go on, if we're lucky.

I persevered and completed my training in Minnesota. Then I worked as an attending at Our Lady of Lourdes Hospital in Camden, New Jersey, and Burlington Memorial Hospital in Mount Holly, New Jersey, for three years. I traveled back to Massachusetts in 1988 and started Fairlawn Rehabilitation Hospital, on that same year, in Worcester. The circle was completing. Sometime after this, I was divorced.

A little later, I remember always holding onto walls while walking. The gait ataxia was getting worse, but what could I do? After this, I used crutches. Unfortunately, I suffered several falls and had to use a scooter to get around the hospital. Again, I persevered, though it was difficult.

I developed another problem around 1992 or so: severe spinal spasticity. My feet would dorsiflex, the knees would flex, and the hips would bend up to my chest every fifteen seconds, especially if I yawned, sneezed, or had to blow my nose. My feet would not touch the floor without the legs flexing up.

I had to be out of work. For the first time, I *couldn't* work. My home physical therapist tried to keep me stretched out to avoid contractures, but unfortunately it was unsuccessful and just resulted in a lot of pain. The spasticity also made all activities of daily living (ADLs) impossible. Life at that time was miserable.

I was quite lucky when I was referred to a neurosurgeon at Boston University Hospital. He had trained in a new procedure which was being developed at St. Luke's Medical Center in Chicago. It involved treating spinal cord–injured and multiple-sclerosis patients with severe spinal spasticity not responsive to oral medications.

It was an Intrathecal Baclofen pump, which was placed subdermally in the left lower quadrant of the abdomen. A tube was placed through my body into the spinal cord, where the liquid Baclofen was to be delivered. The Baclofen was delivered by injecting it with a needle into a port in the pump. The dosage I needed determined how often the injection would be repeated. The proper dose was monitored by a computer. I was fortunate because I was one of the first patients who underwent the procedure; the FDA had not yet approved it. So I was a bit of a willing, but very desperate, guinea pig.

Before the surgery, I had been taking ninety mg of oral Baclofen each day, with no results. I had also tried Dantrium and Valium, both of which would only make me very sleepy but now I at least had relief from the frequent, horrible spasms. Luckily, I responded to the new procedure. I had my life back, though I had to go through a lot of painful but necessary physical therapy in the rehabilitation unit at Boston University Hospital—necessary because, by then, I had developed thirty-degree flexion contractures of both knees.

The therapy involved lying on my stomach with weights on my legs. I also developed an ileus and spent some time with a nasogastric tube. That was in August to September of 1992.

In 1993, I was on large doses of steroids (1,000 mg for five days) during many hospital admissions. In late 1993, I was having some gynecological problems, so I had a D&C, spent more time in an MRI, had to have two uterine ablations, and suffered *another* ileus.

In 1994, I continued taking steroids, in an effort to stabilize the disease, and suffered a bad exacerbation consisting of a cervical (C3) myelopathy. So, no longer responding to steroids, I was started on Interferon Beta-1B (BETASERON). When this didn't seem to be of much help, I was then switched to Beta-1A (AVONEX) in early 1998.

In 1995, I had my first Indiana Pouch, which is a continent urinary diversion made from the ascending colon. This was needed because I had tried the crede technique, intermittent catheterization, a suprapubic catheter, and a Foley without much success. The problem was that I had a dyssynergic, spastic bladder. Even Ditropan stopped helping. I also had my share of infections. Along with this lengthy surgery, I received a hysterectomy and appendectomy and, of course, suffered *yet another* ileus.

In early 1996, a second revision of the Indiana Pouch was done to correct its placement on the abdomen. Immediately following the revision, there was a bowel obstruction, a pneumothorax due to a central line placement—necessary total parenteral nutrition (TPN) because of a continued NG tube—and then placement of a G tube. It was sometime around this time that I had a portacath inserted, because my veins were no longer accessible, most likely due to the many surgeries.

Early in 1998, a second Baclofen pump needed to be done to replace its batteries. Later in 1998, a bilateral salpingo-oophorectomy—the surgical removal of the Fallopian tubes and the ovaries—was necessary, followed by a Pseudomonas-arugenosa infection in the blood, which needed some dangerous IV antibiotics, with many potential side effects.

In late 1998, I had a third revision of the Indiana Pouch done, because the stoma was closing up, making catheterization quite difficult.

In 2001, a third intrathecal Baclofen pump was placed.

The fall of 2003 found me starting on Copaxone. Sometime before this, I had also tried intravenous immunoglobulin (IVIG) therapy and the medication CellCept, but nothing seemed to help stabilize the disease.

Small cataracts and stomach ulcers developed, presumably due to steroids. As luck would have it, the continued steroid use also became ineffective. Shingles on the back was an additional problem, due to immunosuppression.

Atrial fibrillation occurred in 2007 and, for this I was started on Coumadin, until I underwent a successful cardioversion to bring me back into sinus rhythm.

Then I started to have trouble with swallowing and aspiration. It also seemed to be complicated by weakness in the respiratory muscles, due to the multiple sclerosis.

In early 2007, I had a second pneumonia, was treated in the ICU, and needed a ventilator. After suffering a collapsed right lung and yet *another* pneumonia, I agreed to a tracheotomy in the summer of 2007. After all, I was **too often** in ICUs on vents, in respiratory failure.

At this time, I was given a Passy-Muir valve, which allows the passage of air up over the vocal cords, resulting in normal speech.

After failing to pass modified-barium swallowing tests after three trials, I started on continuous tube feedings each night.

In May of 2008, I had an episode of hemoptysis—the coughing-up of blood—but neither the CT nor a bronchoscopy determined the origin of the bleeding.

In June of 2008, I underwent surgery to remove painful scar tissue from the tracheotomy.

In early November 2008, the Baclofen pump was removed again because its batteries needed to be replaced. Later in that same month, surgical excision of the now extremely painful granuloma tissue became necessary. It had again grown around the tracheotomy. The body just does not like this foreign object and hopefully more granuloma tissue won't grow.

For a while, I used a home ventilator. I still take tube feedings by a bolus method three times daily. While I admit that this is not a tasty diet, it certainly is better than being in an ICU battling another pneumonia.

Currently I'm happily free from the ventilator—the machine that has saved my life multiple times. For now I hope that the multiple sclerosis will give me a rest and be stable. Tomorrow will be another day, hopefully a good one. Yet, the future is always unknown with this disease.

Indeed, it's always unknown: as it happens, recently I slipped out of my wheelchair and due to the osteoporosis, I sustained numerous fractures. Not only did I fracture my right hip, I also broke both tibias, fibulas, and ankles.

When you think that everything that could happen has happened, it's best to think again. One morning I could not be woken up by my CNA. She called 911 and the ambulance, the police, and the firemen came to the house. She tells me now that I was taken off by the ambulance and, at some point, suffered two grand mal seizures. I lapsed into a coma and was admitted to the medical ICU at UMass University Hospital.

It was later found that I was septic due to VRE (vancomycin-resistant enterococcus) and pneumonia due to Pseudomonas-arugenosa. Yes, I was once again the victim of two very bad infections.

I remember hearing and recognizing the voices of my CNAs in the hospital room, but I was unable to open my eyes, speak, or lift up my arms no matter how hard I tried. But I knew that I would be okay when I heard the doctor telling everyone that I would be okay.

When I think about it, it's amazing to realize how well my brain was working...thank God.

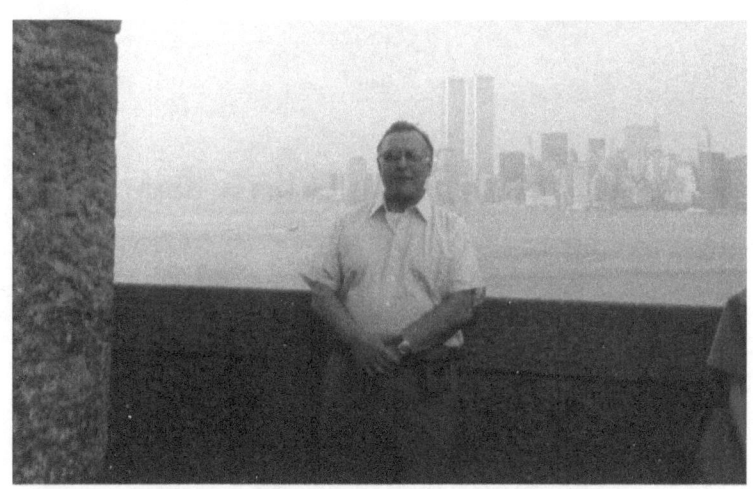

The Author's father standing in front of the World Trade Center.

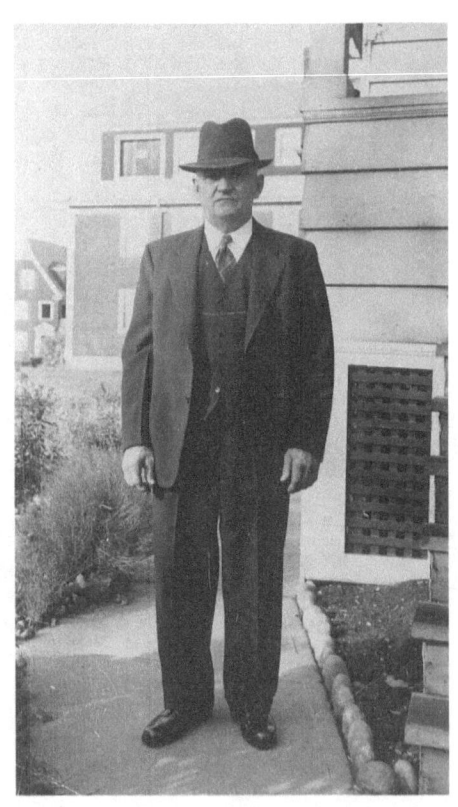

GBC next to his home in Worcester, MA

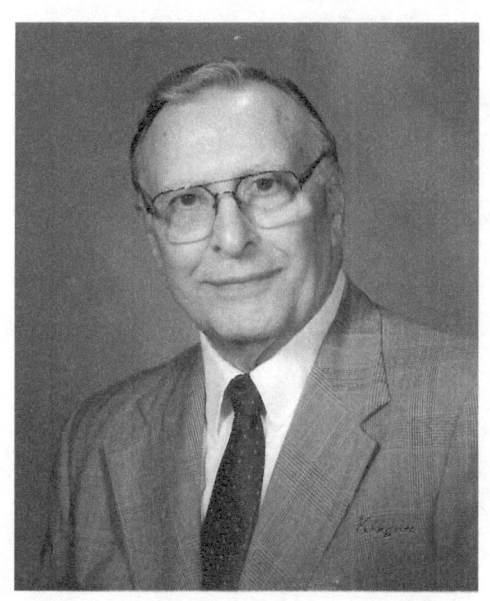

The Author's father in 1992

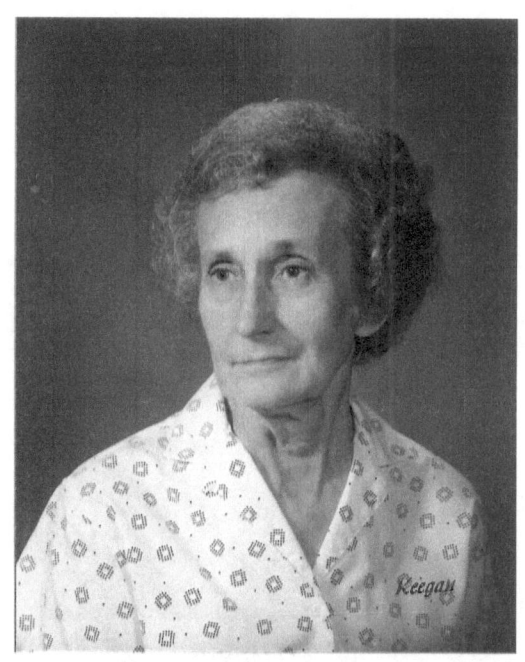

The Author's mother in 1992

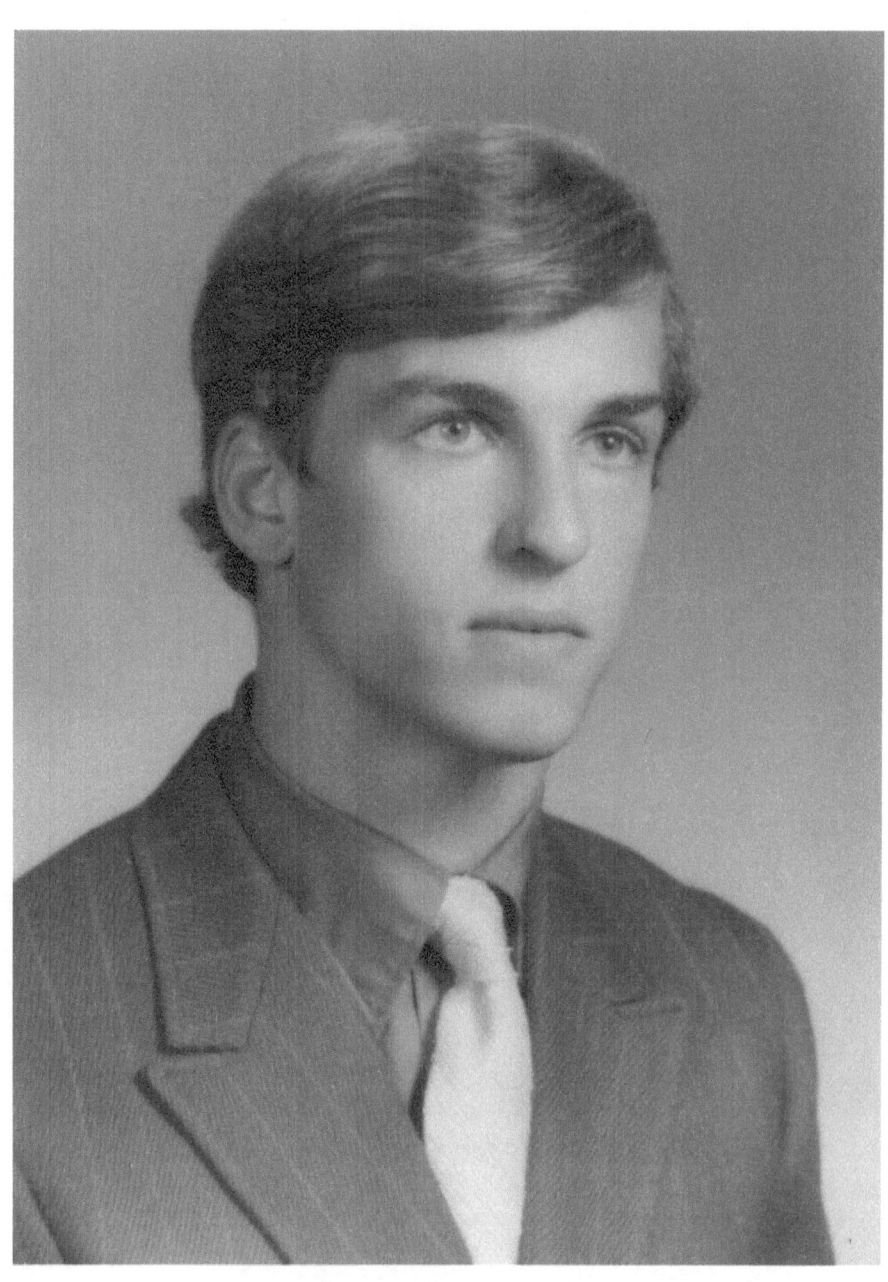

Brother's high-school graduation circa 1970

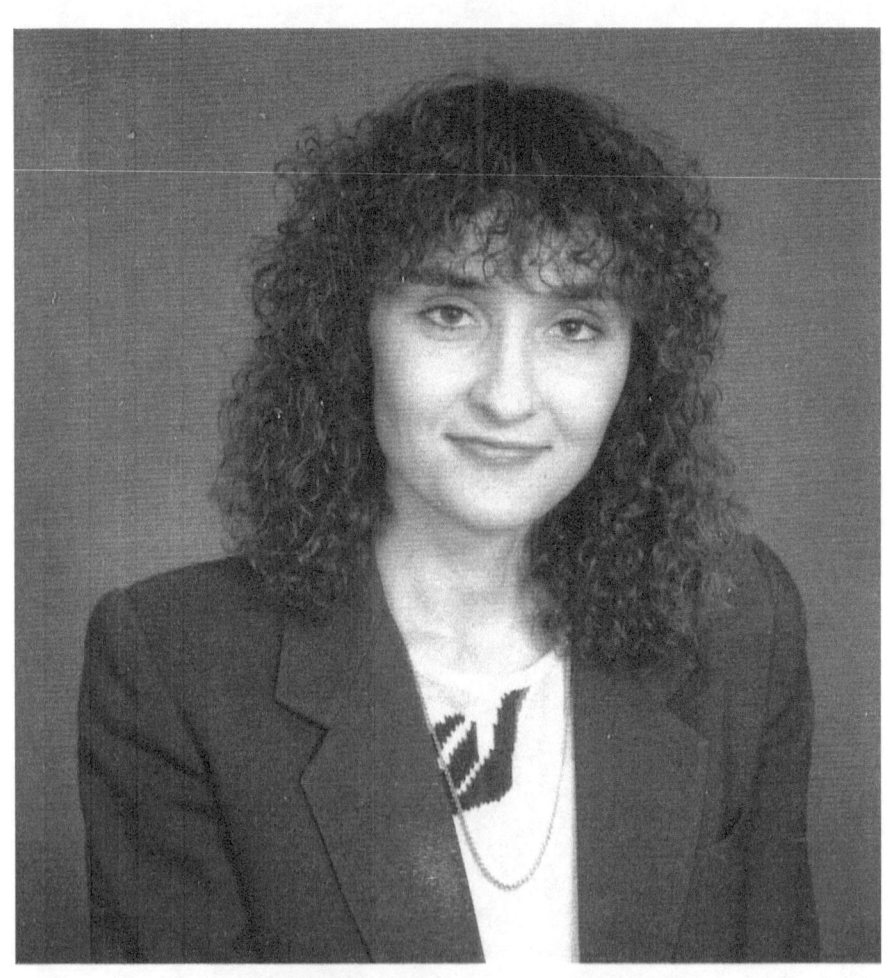

The author circa 2000, while practicing in MA

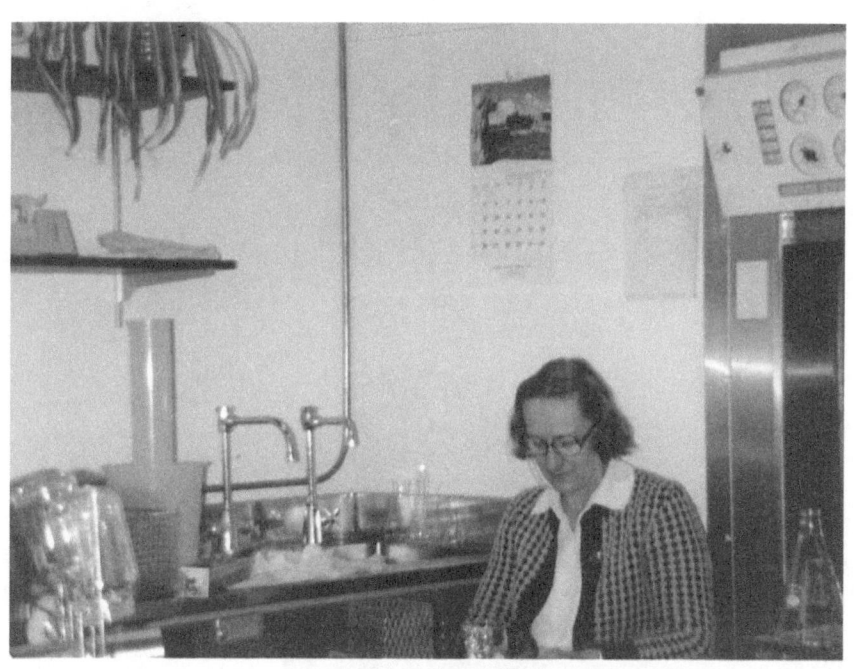

The Author's mother in a lab

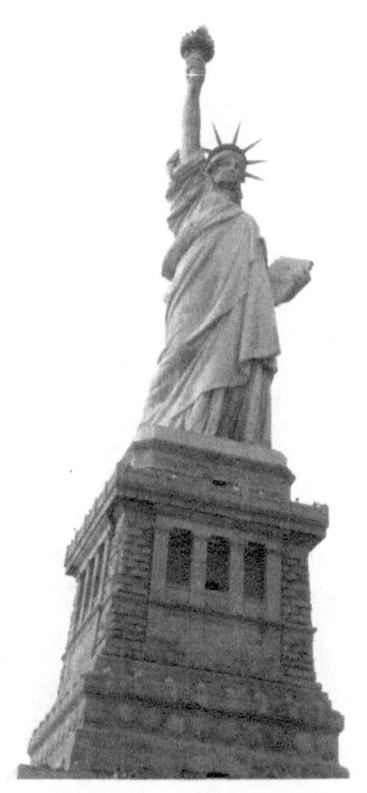

The Statue of Liberty welcoming my grandfather

MULTIPLE SCLEROSIS SYMPTOMS

Now, I'll proceed with discussions of some symptoms in multiple sclerosis:

VISION

NYSTAGMUS

Nystagmus is an oscillation, or rather fast movement in a rhythmic pattern, of the eyeballs, which results in the vision jumping quickly side to side or up and down. This may be one symptom involved in a flare of the disease. In this case, treatment with steroids may be helpful, but I've found that the nystagmus may slowly resolve on its own...or it may not. It may be helpful to find a "window" in the field of vision which is steady, avoiding the extreme directions, and then this can be tolerable.

RETROBULBAR or OPTIC NEURITIS

Optic neuritis occurs when the optic nerve undergoes demyelination. Signals to the visual area of the brain are blocked. The symptom is the sudden loss of vision. I've usually experienced that loss as a white fog wherever I looked. I was unable to see any object, though one time I saw a black space wherever I looked. This was more frightening than usual. This, in combination with lack of good sensation in my hands, made me feel as though I was losing touch with my environment. My usual attempt to keep turning my head to gain sight of everything didn't seem to work as well as usual. The darkness was hard to ignore.

The other bothersome symptom was severe pain in the eye when just looking or applying any slight pressure to it. I hate to recall it, but the optic neuritis has happened several times in both eyes. This, in addition to numbness in the hands, can make functioning very difficult.

My problem with the optic neuritis was usually preceded by stress or a bladder infection. Treatment has been successful with high-dose IV steroids.

CATARACTS

Some medications such as high-dose steroids can have side effects such as cataracts. I've been fortunate, though, because I've needed the steroids many times, have very small cataracts, and no significant visual problems secondary to them. So for me, the benefits of the steroids have outweighed the risks. This benefit/risk ratio is something very important and should be discussed with one's doctor when necessary.

BLURRED VISION

A change in visual acuity which may manifest as a blurring of vision might, again, be a side effect of a medication, but more likely it is a symptom brought on by stress, increased environmental temperature, or infection. It will hopefully resolve with time and cannot usually be improved with glasses. However, I've found the use of my prescription glasses to be beneficial and necessary. Unfortunately, I have to admit that this might also be due to my age (chronological, of course).

DOUBLE VISION

Weakness of the muscles that surround the eyes, so as to provide them stability and movement, causes double vision. These muscles are innervated by cranial nerves from the brainstem, which can also undergo demyelination. There are three cranial nerves supplying eye movement. Number III, IV, and VI move the eyes in all directions. As in other parts of the body, and with other muscles and their respective nerves, demyelination in the area of these cranial nerves causes significant problems by interfering with the passage of the signals carried by the nerves to the muscles, which results in weakness. Thus the eyes cannot move in all of the directions required, in coordination with each other, and double vision results.

This is an annoying, common problem with multiple sclerosis. My experience has been good resolution, again, with the use of high-dose IV steroids. One can also use an eye patch to try to block out some of the conflicting vision.

INTERNUCLEAR OPTHALMOPLEGIA

Internuclear opthalmoplegia occurs when the movement of the eye muscles becomes uncoordinated due to a lesion in the brainstem. The eyes do not move well together, which in turn might result in double vision and can be seen on physical examination.

SWALLOWING

DYSPHAGIA

Dysphagia refers to difficult swallowing. However, with multiple sclerosis it sometimes is not easily determined why or even if it does exist. By this, I mean that patients may deny or not be aware of the difficulty. It is often difficult for the speech therapist to observe an entire meal. Fatigue or too quick of a pace could become an issue toward the end of a meal, and that might affect the swallowing pattern. Of course, the major concern with swallowing is maintaining clarity of the airway.

For this reason, and to determine the proper therapy, a videofluoroscopy of swallowing should be done. This is a study done by a radiologist with a speech therapist in attendance. The therapist prepares various consistencies of food for the patient and the entire swallowing is visualized as it happens.

Some people like me are called "silent aspirators." I have a delayed swallowing reflex and, even though I was aware of the problem, it was not proved until I had a videofluoroscopy done and experienced recurrent pneumonias. You see, when I swallow, the food travels from my mouth to the lungs, instead of the stomach. I also had a problem several times turning the head to the side, when I would become nauseous and vomit in order to avoid aspirating the acidic stomach contents, and thus the resultant pneumonia. Though I spent a good deal of time slurping down thickened liquids and using lemon swabs to quicken and strengthen the swallowing process, this still did not succeed to avoid pneumonia. I tired of the whole issue and decided to not even try electric stimulation, afraid that this, too, would fail.

Thus I ended up with a PEG tube, taking bolus-tube feedings. I've noticed this to be easier and more comfortable than continuous feedings. To date, there have been no side effects.

SPEECH

DYSARTHRIA

Altered speech referred to as dysarthria is another common problem in multiple sclerosis. Again, this is a function dependent on the strength and proper coordination of a number of muscles that control structures such as the lips, tongue, vocal cords, larynx, palate, jaw, and even the lungs.

Once again, demyelination in important areas such as the brainstem and the cerebellum results in disruption of the transmission of nerve signals to the appropriate muscles, and this can result in anything, from slurred, unintelligible speech, to soft, breathy, or harsh and spastic speech patterns. This can become worse with fatigue.

The type of speech will determine the method of therapy chosen by the speech therapist. There are many methods which might be of help.

VERTIGO

The sensation of spinning is vertigo. It can also involve severe nausea and vomiting. It is caused by a lesion in the brainstem, as are visual problems. It can also be caused by inner-ear problems. By now, we are seeing the importance of lesions in the brainstem, a very important structure in the central nervous system.

Whenever I experienced vertigo, I remember being restricted to lying down with a sensation of fluid floating in my head, which would slosh with even my tiniest movement. This was accompanied by severe nausea. At the same time, I was also suffering from double-vision. This was an early exacerbation of the disease for me; at least, that's what I remember. *Disease*...after thirty years, I still can't really get used to that word applying to me.

Treatment for me was successful again with high-dose IV steroids.

MUSCLES

MYOKYMIA

Myokymia is a wormlike twitching of the muscles. I experienced this in a muscle underneath the left eye. I choose to mention this not because it is a common problem in MS, but because this is how MS first appeared in me. In my case, it was a problem because of a lesion in that segment of the brainstem called the pons, where the facial nerve (cranial nerve 7) is located. Myokymia can also be seen in a brainstem glioma, which is a type of cancer. So, at the time of its appearance in me, I prayed to God that my family would not have to witness me dying of a brainstem tumor. I wanted a diagnosis of MS. It persisted for quite a while, before disappearing with the use of some low-dose oral steroids. Even now, it will occasionally reappear with fatigue or stress.

WEAKNESS

As in other situations and other chronic diseases, weakness of muscles is an important problem. It can be a major factor in decreased mobility and ability to independently perform activities of daily living—ADLs.

Exercises in MS can be safely carried out with the guidance of a qualified physical therapist. Good results can be seen. It should be remembered that an increase in the environment's temperature, the presence of infection, or fatigue that is unique to MS might hamper the results. These important issues should always be remembered.

The other very important factor is the demyelination of nerves, which causes weakness that cannot be cured simply by exercising.

I have treated many people with MS and have yet to see anyone welcome his or her need for a wheelchair or assistance with ADLs. These people should not be considered failures, nor lazy. Efforts at such an endeavor are sometimes not rewarded with success. It may only be a matter of time before the same fate befalls others with MS, but hopefully not. As a physiatrist, this should be when I would call for help from other members of the rehab team. This certainly is not a time to give up.

I want to take some time to address the problems of contractures of the various joints that may appear. When muscles are weak, contractures of the joints should and can be avoided with simple, passive range-of-motion exercises. Though frowned upon by some as just maintenance therapies, they are absolutely necessary. Serious disabilities can be avoided in the joints of the neck and extremities.

So remember, please, that while these exercises may not result in any significant strength gain, they are **absolutely** necessary.

AMBULATION

This is a necessary function for many reasons. Multiple factors contribute to the achievement of ambulation and resultant mobility and must be taken into consideration. Some of these are adequate muscle strength in the lower extremities, abdomen, and back. In addition, good bone integrity, balance, sensation, and lack of excessive spasticity are necessary.

There are many more factors, however, which should be mentioned. These, of course, depend upon the diagnosis of the person.

Aides are many and need to be prescribed by a qualified physician or therapist. These can vary from a single-point cane to a mechanical wheelchair. Braces may involve the entire leg and even the torso. The point is that this is a complicated subject and needs to be carefully investigated to achieve optimal, realistic, safe mobility for the person.

SPASTICITY

As I've said before, in multiple sclerosis lesions may occur in the brain or spinal cord. These lesions, or areas of demyelination, interfere with the correct passage of signals to the muscles, resulting in different degrees of spasticity. This may be a disabling condition in ALL aspects of life.

Spasticity is a tight, potentially very painful condition that develops when opposing muscles work at the same time. The pain is caused by the forceful contractions of muscles that should be complementing each other, in balance, to produce a smooth, controlled movement. Instead, opposing muscles work at the same time to produce movements which are jerky, uncoordinated, and uncontrolled.

The tone of the muscles is greatly increased and we also see an increase in tendon reflexes. At other times, movement may not even occur and we see only a tight contraction or rigid position. Muscle contractions which are not properly controlled by the nervous system can, again, be incredibly powerful and painful. I cannot stress this enough.

More detailed neurophysiology on spasticity will have to be found in other sources. I have not done the topic justice. At any rate, we end up with incorrect patterns of muscle stimulation. A physical therapist is the rehabilitation team member who can best deal with spasticity.

Spasticity affecting functions such as sitting, standing, walking, and transferring (especially with people who use wheelchairs as a primary means of mobility) should be addressed. The degree of increased tone present will determine the proper therapy needed. And of course, increased tone in certain extensor muscles is needed to facilitate activities such as sitting upright and walking.

I will quickly address some important issues, now, on this confusing subject:

Stretching of tight muscles is a must. At times, depending on the amount of tone present, this has to be aggressive to achieve good orientation of the limbs and the trunk. Muscles most often needing aggressive stretching are the leg muscles, such as the gastrocnemius, quadriceps, hip adductors, hip flexors, and hip abductors. The back and neck muscles must also be included. The other issue, of course, is contractures of soft tissue, which must be avoided.

With less tone, stretching, while still necessary, can be less forceful and may be accompanied by trials of icing. Theoretically, icing may not only help decrease the tone, it may also provide some comfort, though usually temporary.

Other very important exercises are range of motion, which should be done or demonstrated by the therapist. Depending on the amount of tone present, these may be successfully taught to the patient and caretakers so as to afford some degree of independence and responsibility. They may also help with ADLs, which are usually complicated by spasticity. For these, an occupational therapist will be of great help, introducing adaptive equipment.

Other therapies to be tried could involve proper positioning, especially in bed, with the use of ankle/foot splints. The use of braces might also be helpful. These are made of different materials and their specifics will depend on the function desired. One of the more common braces is the ankle-foot orthosis (AFO), used to prevent the deformity that involves the inversion and pointing-down of the foot and retroversion of the knee. This brace mainly assists with walking.

An important benefit of muscle tone which needs to be remembered is that stress exerted by the muscles on the bones will help prevent bone demineralization, as seen in osteoporosis. So I don't, of course, mean to characterize all tone, especially when functionally needed, as unwanted.

Finally, there are some medications that should be mentioned:

The first is Baclofen or Lioresal. This is a common agent in the war against spasticity in multiple sclerosis. The mechanism of action of the drug takes place in the spinal-cord nerves. Since all patients with multiple sclerosis have different degrees of spasticity, different doses will be helpful. The dose needs to be titrated according to the effect achieved and the needs of the patient. While it can successfully reduce spasticity, too much can cause fatigue and very little tone. This can be a functional problem, especially with the muscles of the leg and torso.

I had a great deal of spinal spasticity not treated well with 90 mg of daily oral Baclofen. So, I received an intrathecal Baclofen (Lioresal) pump. This works by delivering a programmed amount of liquid Baclofen directly into the spinal fluid that surrounds the spinal cord. I get my pump refilled every three months. It has been a great help. This therapy should be discussed with the neurologist.

Another drug commonly used to treat spasticity in multiple sclerosis is Dantrium (sodium dantrolene). This works directly on the muscle and, like Lioresal, can have a strong effect, causing weakness and fatigue. Its dosage also needs to be carefully adjusted to the patient's needs. I didn't find this helpful, even when used in conjunction with Valium, which I'll address next.

Valium (diazepam) is a strong medicine that induces sleep, can relax one's anxiety, and may become addictive. Used by some to reduce night spasms, I had no luck, however, with this. It did make me feel very sleepy, but the spasms continued, as did the pain.

There are some other medications available, such as Botox, but the appropriate one needs to be determined by a good physical exam from one's doctor.

SENSATION

I have chosen to address sensory abnormalities because they are so common in MS, and are not only bothersome but also of great concern, evoking much worry. These are caused by demyelination in areas of the brain or spinal cord connecting to the extremities.

TEMPERATURE PERCEPTION and NUMBNESS

These can be other annoying, serious problems with MS. Again, demyelination causes faulty message transmission. Therefore, the ability to accurately distinguish hot from cold or sharp from dull can be difficult.

Of course, the extent of these problems varies from person to person, so the necessary help and monitoring should be offered to avoid accidents involving burns and cuts.

Although very annoying, these problems are not serious enough, nor do they indicate worsening of the disease to warrant treatment with drugs. Numbness may overlap with something called astereognosis, which I'll now address:

ASTEREOGNOSIS

This is also a very bothersome problem. Astereognosis, or loss of stereognosis, is the inability to identify objects on how they feel, without looking at them. It often occurs with numbness, and the two together are disabling and inconvenient. Again, there is faulty signal transmission somewhere between the brain and the hands due to demyelination.

An example often used in an evaluation by an occupational therapist will be to see if the patient can distinguish different coins from each other; or the person might be asked to correctly identify objects such as a pencil or a pen, or even smaller objects such as paper clips, nuts, or screws.

Just experiencing this problem, though it is quite concerning and annoying, warrants no medicinal treatment.

PARESTHESIAS

Paresthesias are common and seen in many people with MS, as well as in others without the disease. Once again, the problem is due to demyelination interfering with signals from the brain and spinal cord to the extremities.

They are often described as a burning, tingling, or prickling sensation. It is normally felt after continued pressure has been applied to a nerve commonly in a limb such as at the elbow or in a leg after crossing the knees.

In MS, it can be a more sustained sensation. Many people with MS have told me that, in retrospect, they remember paresthesias long before they were diagnosed.

These bothersome issues should resolve subtly on their own, just as they appeared. No treatment is needed, but coping is necessary.

TASTE

Taste is an important sensation for all of us. It involves the 7th and 9th cranial nerves in the brainstem. Demyelination of those nerves interferes with signal transmission.

Again, while loss of this sensation is another real bother, it will hopefully resolve quickly on its own. I've experienced this several times, but no treatment was necessary, and it was followed by complete recovery.

PROPRIOCEPTION

Proprioception is a necessary sensation on which we depend to use our extremities. It is present in such organs as muscles, tendons, and joints. Without this sensation, we are unable to use important parts of our bodies, such as our hands. For example, without it, we cannot tell which position our fingers are in.

I've had the awful experience of losing the proprioception in my dominant hand. After this happened, I was unable to write holding a pen. This was because I had no sensory feedback from the muscles and joints in the fingers of the hand. Neither was I able to voluntarily control the movement of the fingers. They would not stop moving on their own, even while I was sleeping. It was as if they were searching for something out in space. In fact, the severity of my fingers' movement is more correctly described as a movement disorder or dystonia, another problem which can occur in MS, and which can also lead to contractures of the joints.

Because my MCP (metacarpophalangeal) joints were all repeatedly extending in a horrible fashion, looking like a "claw" hand, the occupational therapist fabricated a splint for the hand to block the excessive MCP extension. This helped not only to correct the position of the fingers but also with alleviation of the pain.

The first time that this happened, over several months I had a complete remission. Of course, it was only one, albeit the major symptom, in a bad exacerbation for which I received five days of high-dose IV steroids. Unfortunately, this happened several more times. The other hand has also suffered such a loss. Each time it was, of course, complicated by numbness and lack of stereognosis. The recovery has now become less complete.

TREMORS

Tremor is an oscillating movement that can occur in the head, extremities, torso, or even the face, and thus affecting the speech. It is caused by demyelination in the basal ganglia or in the cerebellum, the latter of which makes up the rear of the brain. The cerebellum has connections with other important parts of the central nervous system, including the brainstem and the spinal cord. Coordinated movement results by communicating with these other regions.

There are many different types of tremors. They can be large and very noticeable, with wide oscillations. They may also be only minimal and/or at rest. Others may be with voluntary movements; this is the intention tremor. Some are seen with spasticity; others occur with anxiety. Movements of the trunk, the head, and the jaw may also be affected. And, as with all other symptoms of multiple sclerosis, they are worsened with fatigue.

Tremors are quite disabling and can be difficult to successfully manage. Many different rehabilitation team members must be involved. Speech therapists would be the best to address any speech problems that may be seen; occupational and physical therapists would be able to address tremors involving the head, torso, and extremities.

Exercises involving repetitive motions could be tried in an attempt to retrain the muscles in the extremities, so as to achieve normal, automatic motion. This is based on the "wiring" already present in the nervous system.

Bracing might be useful mainly in the head and torso, but also probably in the extremities. This would, of course, depend on the type of brace proposed and the function desired. Weighting with small wrist or ankle weights could also be tried, in an attempt to inhibit tremors in the extremities.

It should, of course, be mentioned that fatigue with both the repetitive motion exercises and the weights might, on the other hand, adversely affect the results. These activities need to be carefully balanced.

Unfortunately, tremors are difficult problems that I've often seen in my practice and have personally experienced. They appear unexpectedly, and only luck and hard work *may* bring about improvement. There are medications that can be tried, but this information may be found in other sources and should be discussed with one's doctor.

BLADDER

Many people with multiple sclerosis will have, at one time or another, difficulty with bladder control. The difficulty posed by the disease will depend on where the lesion is interfering with signal transmission in the system that controls the bladder.

This system is one that basically involves connection between the bladder, the spinal cord, the brainstem, and the brain. So, one can imagine the number of problems that might occur.

The most common disorder seen with multiple sclerosis is a spastic bladder. This low-volume bladder needs to be emptied frequently, creating "urgency," and should always be emptied completely. This might be more difficult than one would expect.

When the bladder fills to capacity, nerves in the spinal cord signal the bladder muscle to contract, pushing out urine. This usually results in frequency and urgency. The bladder muscle may hypertrophy, or we could say it becomes thickened.

Besides being very disruptive to life, this urgency and frequency result in much anxiety, maybe even dribbling of urine or incontinence. The bathroom is *never too close by!* What is happening is disruption of communication somewhere between the reflex center in the bladder and the brain. It becomes impossible for one to avoid the reflex and voluntarily hold the urine.

This calls for an evaluation to be done by a urologist and should be the beginning of a good relation between an interested, competent physician and an appropriately concerned patient.

Another type of bladder which can be seen in multiple sclerosis is a big-capacity or "lazy," flaccid bladder. This would be when there is faulty communication between the bladder and the brain. Here again, as with the spastic bladder, adequate emptying is the main issue to protect the proper anatomy of the ureters and kidneys, by preventing the backflow of urine.

Finally, there may be what is called a dyssynergic bladder. Here we see an uncoordinated bladder. In this case, contraction of the bladder muscle occurs, while at the same time there is either contraction OR relaxation of the urethral sphincter muscle. Thus, there may be inability to completely void due to a sudden, spastic-bladder contraction AND contraction of the sphincter muscle.

This also leads to trouble holding the urine and may result in dribbling or incontinence...or it might involve the sudden need to void because of a bladder contraction and incontinence due to a relaxed sphincter muscle. A full, flaccid bladder may also result in dribbling or incontinence because of uncoordinated sphincter-muscle activity.

In other words, the situation might become quite complicated and difficult to successfully manage. There are a number of medications that may be tried to control either the forceful contractions of the spastic bladder or the lack of contractions in the flaccid, lazy bladder. These can be tried and the results followed by the urologist.

Techniques which might be tried to afford bladder control are many. Success depends on the specific bladder condition. The first is the Crede maneuver. It involves manually pressing down on the abdomen in the direction of the bladder, in an attempt to completely empty it. This would have to be done at timed intervals or when an urge to empty is felt. Of course, this would be most successful with the flaccid bladder. Residual volumes would have to be checked by catheterization to assure adequate emptying and to avoid infection.

Another technique might be the insertion of a suprapubic catheter, which would be emptied periodically. Intermittent catheterization can also be learned and done at needed intervals, in conjunction—as with all of these techniques—with a fluid schedule. Avoidance of drinking fluids is never a means by which one achieves continence.

A Foley catheter may be another option. The types of catheter available for men and women are different. A leg bag would be needed and also nighttime gravity drainage. The risk of infection is high, because the Foley catheter is a foreign object that can easily introduce bacteria into the urine. The urine should always be kept as free from infection as possible.

Finally, a urinary diversion might be chosen. This is a major operation done by the urologist. There are different types. A continent urinary diversion involves redirecting the urine from the bladder to another storage area. It also means hooking up the ureters to this new storage area (usually a piece of bowel), and then this "bowel," or "neobladder," is catheterized, allowing thus the kidneys to drain. So the bladder would essentially be bypassed, no longer of use in the new system. This is a rather simplistic, incomplete explanation of a complex operation. A much better description could be obtained in a conversation with one's urologist.

Again, medications might also be needed with some of these

techniques. ALL of these techniques must be discussed with the urologist.

As with other parts of the body, infection is possible and must be avoided. Gram-negative organisms are commonly seen in a bladder infection, but gram-positive organisms may also infect the bladder. Instead of trying to quickly describe the microbiology involved, I think it will be more practical to describe what one should look for if a bladder infection, or UTI (urinary-tract infection), is suspected.

Common findings in a bladder infection would be darker color of the urine, maybe even a foul odor, or perhaps specks of blood. Of course, increased urgency or frequency, burning, and increase in oral temperature could also be seen.

People with chronic conditions may experience an increase in the symptoms of their disease. These signs and symptoms should **not** be ignored and consultation with one's doctor should follow. A sterile "as possible" urine sample is obtained for two basic tests: a urinalysis, and if this shows bacteria, a culture of the urine is done to identify the organisms and the appropriate antibiotic. The ENTIRE course of antibiotics should follow.

BOWEL

Again, as with the bladder, most people with multiple sclerosis will have problems with bowel control from time to time. The digestive system is a set of organs also controlled by the nervous system. So, areas of demyelination interfere with signal transmission and normal function.

Constipation can be a problem for many people with multiple sclerosis. Lack of muscle strength may result in immobility, which in turn will interfere with normal passage of stool. A voluntary decrease in fluid, in an attempt to manage the bladder, will also inhibit good bowel function. This results in hard stool, also difficult to pass.

The issue of a proper diet is, of course, very important, but also varies somewhat from person to person. Good rules, though, would be to include fruits (prepared to one's liking and any dietary or swallowing restrictions); vegetables (also keep in mind any necessary restrictions); and necessary fiber.

So as you see, I have not offered a "cookbook" of rules, because everyone does have his or her own needs, and I would recommend consulting a dietician or asking one's doctor to address the problem more specifically. There are also many medications which may be of help.

Diarrhea can also be a problem in multiple sclerosis, but is less common than constipation. Reflex action of the bowel or side effects of medications such as antibiotics may be the cause. Trying to bulk up the stool might help. Again, I would suggest asking your doctor for help... and be persistent! Once you meet with success, stick with it.

SKIN

Skin problems may result because of continued pressure over a bony prominence or area of soft tissue. This is complicated by the person's lack of sensation in the area, inability to rise up off the area due to weakness, or incontinence of bladder or bowel.

Continued pressure results in blockage of necessary blood flow. Skin problems first appear as a red area that does not "blanche," or turn to normal skin tone with pressure, and which then returns to the red color. This means that blood is not actively flowing in that area. Ischemia, or tissue death, may already be occurring. This is time for intervention in order to prevent more damage.

There are many different types of possible therapies for compromised skin. I won't try to list them all, because each breakdown is different and needs different treatment. Many times, the caretaker will have more experience and success with a certain therapy on a particular breakdown, and so this might determine the appropriate choice.

The use of proper padding under all areas at risk should occur. Padded foam, jell cushions are good for wheelchair users and alternating air-pressure mattresses are appropriate for beds. Tegaderm can be used for heels and any other areas as a translucent dressing to mainly provide protection from sheer forces, while allowing observation of the skin condition. Duoderm is another dressing which can be helpful with skin breakdown that is further advanced.

I've addressed these issues mainly for people who are weak and more susceptible to skin breakdown. Proper therapy will depend on the degree of damage that has occurred. Good nutrition should also be included.

It's important to remember that bony prominences such as the back of the head, the elbows, the shoulder blades, the bottom of the spine (sacrum), and the heels need to be monitored. This is when the person is lying on his or her back.

Side-lying calls for attention to the shoulders, elbows, hips, knees, and the sides of the ankle joints. When lying on the side, pillows should be placed between the legs for comfort and relief of contact between the knees and the ankles.

An important thing to remember is that damaging pressure to the skin can involve the tissues beneath, including the muscles and bones. If this is seen, it calls for much more complicated and immediate therapy. The skills of a surgeon might be needed. We could be talking about removal of dead tissue (debridement), different types of dressings (such as wet to dry), or even skin flaps.

Another important issue is the prevention of infection. This definitely needs to be successfully treated. Continued observation is also mandatory.

While sheer stress or continued pressure can be very damaging, even simple things—like lying down on wrinkled bed sheets or other items for a long time—can begin to destroy tissue.

Finally, it is important to remember that bedsores, or decubiti, which we've been talking about, are like icebergs. By this, I mean that most of the pathology or diseased tissue is beneath the surface of the skin. So, don't be fooled by the surface appearance. More damage may be lurking underneath. Beware always!

PAIN

In multiple sclerosis, pain is not uncommon. I have experienced it myself and have had many patients complain of sensations described as burning, tingling, aching, throbbing, or sharp.

I remember the awful pain from the spasticity, which felt as if the muscles were being ripped from the bones. Or there may be discomfort described as if one is being squeezed around the torso. Nociceptive input from the extremities is perceived as obnoxious sensation by the brain.

The many strange sensations that are experienced by people with multiple sclerosis sometimes seem to defy simple explanations, but it is reasonable to blame them on lesions between the brain and the spinal cord, interfering with signal transmission. Difficult to describe, yet very real, these sensations are often hard to diagnose and to be treated to the patient's satisfaction.

Any complaint of pain should, of course, be respected, worked up as needed, and attempts made to treat it. Pain can be very disabling. There are many medications available, but one needs to be cautious to avoid sedation or addiction. There are always side effects, as with the nonsteroidals, which might bring on more problems. Again, a good physical exam is always needed and sometimes imaging with CT scans and MRIs is warranted.

Both personally and professionally, I've found few medications to be of help, though there are some good options for specific needs. Diversion with hobbies; trips to a new or favorite location; meditation, yoga, acupuncture, massage, or tai chi for some; or other exercises, as recommended by a good physical therapist, may help.

Goals would be to keep fit; maintain painless movement in the extremities; reduce spasticity, if present; and increase one's independence with ADLs. I would NOT recommend manipulation of the spine. Consultation with someone who specializes in pain management may also help.

FATIGUE

Overwhelming fatigue can be very common in multiple sclerosis. It is often associated with difficulty to sleep due to painful night spasms. Other factors might be stress, overextending oneself physically, weakness due to increased environmental temperature, or illness such as an infection.

Again, demyelination in tracts of the central nervous system and indirectly in the peripheral nervous system may be part of the causative factor. Appropriate treatments may involve sleep medication prescribed by one's doctor. Spasms are also manageable according to their severity, response to medications, and physical therapy.

Conservation of energy is also a key factor. Help with this important step can be provided by an occupational therapist. ALL multiple-sclerosis patients should be aware of the damaging effect of increased environmental temperatures.

Cool surroundings, avoidance of humidity, and use of air conditioning are a must. Of course, infections—whether in the urine, lungs, skin, or blood—must be appropriately treated.

INSURANCE

I want to encourage you to purchase a good insurance plan that you might need before the MS worsens. Any government-sponsored health insurance, like Medicare, should also have an adequate secondary plan. Don't forget to apply for Social Security disability and any disability from your workplace. Good luck with life insurance, because MS is a bad diagnosis to put on an application. And don't miss paying any premiums!

MULTIPLE SCLEROSIS MEDICATIONS

This will be a short summary of some medications now frequently used in multiple sclerosis. I recommend that one ask one's neurologist for complete information on each drug. These explanations have been simplified.

AVONEX (Interferon Beta-1A)

Avonex is given by IM (an injection into the muscle) once a week. Composed of amino acids, the "building blocks" of protein, it exerts antiviral and some other quite complicated effects. The drug's mechanism of action in multiple sclerosis has not been completely defined.

Appropriate for use in people with relapsing-remitting multiple sclerosis, it has proven to reduce the number of exacerbations and to slow down the disability process. Potential side effects are many, but it is quite tolerable.

REBIF (Interferon Beta-1A)

Rebif is an interferon injected subdermally **three times a week**. It's used in people with relapsing-remitting MS so as to decrease the number of flare-ups and their disability results therein.

BETASERON (Interferon Beta-1B)

Betaseron is another interferon which is injected subdermally **every other day**. Also used mainly in people with relapsing-remitting multiple sclerosis, it has also been proven to reduce the number of exacerbations. Again, its mechanism of action in multiple sclerosis is not yet well understood. Its side effects are much like those with Avonex and are also tolerable. As with other protein compounds, antibodies may develop resistance to the drug, thereby try to limit its use.

COPAXONE (Glatiramer Acetate Injection)

Copaxone is composed of four amino acids and is injected into the subcutaneous tissue **every day**. It is used in people with relapsing-remitting multiple sclerosis so as to reduce the number of exacerbations. Though its mechanism of action is not fully understood, it is successful in reducing the number of flare-ups of the disease. It may also have many side effects, though again it is usually quite tolerable.

IVIG (Immunoglobulin)

Administered intravenously, IVIG has components equivalent to human plasma. Testing is carried out in this compound in order to protect against the transmission of several diseases to the recipient. Its importance is in its ability to supply antibodies to the recipient.

I remember receiving this by the intravenous route, while the nurse had to carefully monitor the blood pressure and other vitals. It's a very expensive therapy, as are all of the other multiple-sclerosis medications. It is successful in some people.

PREDNISONE

Acute attacks are often treated with corticosteroids (such as prednisone), to decrease the inflammation in the area of demyelination and to shorten the exacerbation. Though improvement cannot be guaranteed, at least one can hope to return to one's baseline. Sometimes this happens.

I think there may be some psychological benefits here as well. However, there are a number of side effects all too often seen with this medication. That is why the dosage is usually quickly tapered.

CELLCEPT

CellCept is a powerful immunosuppressive drug normally used to keep transplant (kidney, heart, lung, and liver) recipients from rejecting their transplanted organs. This medicine may be taken orally as a pill. Its side effects may be the development of certain cancers, such as lymphomas, or serious infections. This calls for careful monitoring by the physician.

TYSABRI

This is a medication given by infusion for people with relapsing-remitting multiple sclerosis. It is used to slow the all-too-often problem of worsening disability in multiple sclerosis and the number of flare-ups. It may be used in people who have not responded adequately to the other multiple-sclerosis medications.

Unfortunately, Tysabri increases the risk of progressive multifocal leukoencephalopathy (PML). This is a rare brain infection which can cause worsening disability and even be fatal. There is no known treatment or cure for PML. It is not even known who would be affected by PML, why or when. Again, this medication must be carefully monitored.

INVESTIGATIONAL THERAPIES:

Ongoing research includes Chronic Cerebrospinal Venous Insufficiency (CCSVI), which is being introduced by Dr. Paolo Zamboni, from the University of Ferrara in Italy. In addition, researchers are investigating the therapeutic use of vitamin D in humans and Resveratrol in animals. Furthermore, many types of stem-cell research are under way.

Dr. Paolo Zamboni, from the University of Ferrara in Italy, has identified Chronic Cerebrospinal Venous Insufficiency, or CCSVI. Zamboni reported that this is abnormal blood drainage caused by narrowed veins in the neck. When treated with balloon angioplasty (in a new way), the MS symptoms improve.

In addition, Dr. Colleen Hayes has found that vitamin D made by cells in the skin, after exposure to sunlight, may suppress the immune response seen in MS. In 2010, Dr. Ellen Mowry reported an inverse finding in the level of vitamin D found in the blood of children and adolescents with subsequent relapses.

Resveratrol, a natural component found in red wine, was investigated by Dr. Ikuo Tsunoda to see if nerve cells might be protected from damage when treated by this constituent. He reported a reduced mortality in treated mice, which might be attributed to nerve protection.

Dr. Dimitrios Karussis treated mice with adult mesenchymal stem cells, which are seen in human bone marrow and fat, and found that the nerve fibers were left intact when compared to untreated mice (the controls).

When an adult mouse's neural stem cells are injected into the blood or brain cavities of mice with EAE (an MS-like disease), Doctors Stefano Pluchino and Gianvito Martino found that these cells move throughout the brain and spinal cord to areas of tissue damage, and by repairing myelin, they help reverse clinical disease.

Along with his team, Dr. Steven A. Goldman found that transplanting OPCs (oligodendrocyte precursor cells) into mice that don't make myelin results in an almost complete restoration of their lost neurological function.

Altering gene activity in Schwann cells, which are good at repairing lost myelin in the arms and legs of the body's periphery but not in the central nervous system (CNS), is being investigated by Dr. Anne Baron-Van Evercooren. She is looking at the ability of these altered cells to migrate into lesion sites of the CNS and carry out their repair activities in mice.

So, you see, with these doctors and their ongoing research, there is a lot of hope.

EPILOGUE

At this time, yes, I use a wheelchair for mobility. The weakness of the legs, along with the lack of good sensation, the spasticity, *and* the osteoporosis, all of it has left me with no alternative. The hands have developed tremors; spasticity is now present here, too; and the lack of good sensation has, likewise, unfortunately become a major issue. The eyes are currently affected by blurred vision, along with horizontal and vertical nystagmus.

My house has been expanded to make it wheelchair-accessible. I need to use the town's wheelchair vans for transportation. I am still licensed, board-certified, and live hoping that, **some day,** there may be a medicine that can change this situation.

Though I've certainly had my share of problems, each morning that I wake up and realize I am still alive and not acutely ill is another day that I've been given. I've learned that multiple sclerosis can make it extremely difficult to plan for the next day, and that no tomorrow is guaranteed. Therefore, I try to make the best of each day. Even though sometimes I don't feel like I'm up to another challenge, life does go on… and so, I'd like to also encourage you to take advantage of every day. There's a reason that you're still here, so don't give up!

Now, I'd like to end by citing a line from Dylan Thomas: "Do not go gently into that good night." I hope that you can find meaning in this statement. For me, this means to not give up the struggle, even if I must change my strategy to keep going as the disease progresses. I'll keep trying to deal with my potentially devastating problem, for I don't know of any chronic disease that isn't devastating. We need to remember that life is an important gift we've been given, and it should be cherished. It makes sense to do our best and to hopefully profit from our efforts. As hard as it is at times, it's a good feeling to have others marvel at how we manage to keep our spirits up, despite many difficulties.

I hope that this book has encouraged you to do just that.

I want to humbly thank you for the time and patience you've invested in reading this brief summary of multiple sclerosis. Hopefully, it has been helpful. My best wishes to you and yours in the future, and may God bless you.

BIBLIOGRAPHY

I owe a good review of my knowledge to the following authors, their books, editors, and publishers (special thanks also go to my editor, Maria Fernandes-Jaeger, of Eagle Eye Editorial Services, in New York City):

Evercooren, Anne Baron-Van et al., cited in *National MS Society Magazine*, Summer 2010: *Brain*, Vol. 133, 2010, 406–20.

Goldman, Steven A. and Ian D. Duncan, cited in *National MS Society Magazine*, Summer 2010: *Cell Stem Cell*, Vol. 2, 2008, 553–65.

Hayes, Colleen et al., "Vitamin D May Suppress the Immune Response Involved in MS," *The Journal of Immunology*, Vol. 183, 2009, 3672–81.

Karussis, Dimitrios, cited in *National MS Society Magazine*, Summer 2010: *Archives of Neurology*, Vol. 65, 2008, 753–61.

Mowry, Ellen, "Vitamin D Status Is Associated with Relapse Rate in Pediatric-Onset MS," Annals of Neurology Online, Vol. 67, 618–24, University of California, San Francisco, Accepted January, 2010, http://www3.interscience.wiley.com/journal/123246501/abstract.

Pluchino, Stefano and Gianvito Martino, cited in *National MS Society Magazine*, Summer 2010: *Nature*, Vol. 422, 2003, 688–94.

Schapiro, Randall T., *Multiple Sclerosis: A Rehabilitation Approach to Management*, Vol. 4, Demos Publications, New York, NY, 1991.

Scheinberg, Labe C. (ed.), *Multiple Sclerosis: A Guide for Patients and Their Families*, 2nd Printing. Raven Press, New York, NY, 1984.

Sinaki, Mehrsheed (ed.), *Basic Clinical Rehabilitation Medicine*. B.C. Decker Inc., Philadelphia, PA, 1987.

Tsunoda, Ikuo, "Resveratrol and MS," cited in *National MS Society Magazine*, Summer 2010, "World Congress of MS 2008," Abstract, p. 212.

Zamboni, Paolo, "Chronic Cerebrospinal Venous Insufficiency in Patients with Multiple Sclerosis," cited in *National MS Society Magazine*, Summer 2010, *Journal of Neurology Neurosurgery & Psychiatry*, Vol. 80, 2009, 392–99.

www.ingramcontent.com/pod-product-compliance
Lightning Source LLC
Chambersburg PA
CBHW021253280526
45784CB00005B/2350